FINDING FAITH THROUGH FIBROMYALGIA

Marian ~
Life - it's
all about
Jesus!

Sue
Schmidt

Finding Faith Through Fibromyalgia

a woman's journey

SUE SCHMIDT

Tate Publishing & *Enterprises*

Finding Faith Through Fibromyalgia
Copyright © 2010 by Sue Schmidt. All rights reserved.

No part of this publication may be reproduced, stored in a retrieval system or transmitted in any way by any means, electronic, mechanical, photocopy, recording or otherwise without the prior permission of the author except as provided by USA copyright law.

All scripture quotations, unless otherwise indicated, are taken from the Holy Bible, New International Version®. NIV®. Copyright © 1973, 1978, 1984 by International Bible Society. Used by permission of Zondervan. All rights reserved.

This book is designed to provide accurate and authoritative information with regard to the subject matter covered. This information is given with the understanding that neither the author nor Tate Publishing, LLC is engaged in rendering legal, professional advice. Since the details of your situation are fact dependent, you should additionally seek the services of a competent professional.

The opinions expressed by the author are not necessarily those of Tate Publishing, LLC.

Published by Tate Publishing & Enterprises, LLC
127 E. Trade Center Terrace | Mustang, Oklahoma 73064 USA
1.888.361.9473 | www.tatepublishing.com

Tate Publishing is committed to excellence in the publishing industry. The company reflects the philosophy established by the founders, based on Psalm 68:11,
"The Lord gave the word and great was the company of those who published it."

Book design copyright © 2010 by Tate Publishing, LLC. All rights reserved.
Cover design by Chris Webb
Interior design by Stephanie Woloszyn

Published in the United States of America

ISBN: 978-1-61663-777-4
1. Health & Fitness / Diseases / General   2. Religion / Faith
10.07.13

ACKNOWLEDGEMENTS

Julie Edman: thank you for your honesty in needing spiritual help instead of just information on fibromyalgia at our support group meetings. God used you to plant the seed for this book.

Julie, Marci, Marilyn and Diana: you are my support group. Thank you for your encouragement at each month's meetings.

Iva: thank you for proofreading and for your friendship. Becky: thank you also for proofreading.

Gabe and Becky: My two terrific children. You both love the Lord and you both chose terrific Christian spouses Beth and Evan. I've been a mom for twenty-nine years and I'm still in awe that God chose me to be your mom. I love you all very much.

Rick: You have been my constant faithful friend and husband. You are so generous with your time and ready to take over without hesitation whenever I haven't been able to. You are on this fibromyalgia journey with me and you have never complained. You have always been understanding of my condition. You have been such a blessing in my life. I love you.

Naomi: Mom, thank you for wanting me, caring for me and guiding me to the Lord.

God: you needed to remove all distraction from my life before I could hear you calling me to be your servant. What a privilege. Thank you for writing this book through me. I don't have the words to describe what an awesome experience this has been to see your hand so clearly at work.

Tate Publishing: thank you for believing in me and for giving me the opportunity to spread the message God wants others to hear.

This book is dedicated to all people who live with daily pain no matter the form, that they may know Jesus as their Savior.

Table of Contents

Forward	11
Chapter 1: Healing	19
Chapter 2: Weakness	33
Chapter 3: Nourishment	47
Chapter 4: Joy	61
Chapter 5: Forgetfulness	73
Chapter 6: Forgiveness	83
Epilogue	103

Finding Faith through Fibromyalgia

Foreword

In 2004 I began noticing fatigue and "traveling" pain. One day the pain and stiffness would be in my hips, the next day my back and the day after that in my shoulders. The pain was usually accompanied with headaches, which could be severe. After several months of experiencing this abnormality I thought I had good reason to see a specialist. I made an appointment with a rheumatologist in 2005 who diagnosed me with fibromyalgia.

It's been estimated there are 10 million Americans who have been diagnosed with fibromyalgia. I am one of them. With so many afflicted, one would think fibromyalgia was common knowledge; it isn't. I had just learned how to pronounce the word. I felt stunned by the number of questions, none of which had answers, and the feeling of being totally alone. I told no one, keeping it to myself for the next few years. How could I explain what I knew nothing about? My rheumatologist handed me a single tri fold brochure with minimal information. To top it off I was no longer able to do my stressful physically demanding job.

After three years of hiding and dealing with the unanswered questions, I began to feel the need for a support group. I contacted a couple friends who knew other people with fibromyalgia and our group began to evolve. We came together that first meeting in September 2008 with the following goals: to offer encouragement, share knowledge and educate one another on exercise, diet and supplements.

My goal was to keep the group small to give us a chance to get to know one another and feel more open to helping one another on a personal level. The lessons I prepared began with the basics: What is fibromyalgia and its symptoms? How do you deal with the diagnosis? How can your loved ones support you? From there we went onto guest speakers.

Once the lesson is concluded and the carafes are full of coffee we visit about our lives or ask, "Have you also been experiencing this pain because it's new for me?" We have grown from five strangers into five friends.

How I have longed for Jesus' healing in my life. I didn't realize it then but I had already received his healing, which came in the form of spiritual healing.

Paul, imprisoned for spreading the Good News of Jesus Christ, authored many books of the Bible from jail. My particular favorite is Philippians. Philippians, which is found in the New Testament, has 104 verses filled with encouragement and joy. Paul states in chapter one, verse 12 (NIV), "that what has happened to me has really served to advance the gospel. As a result it has become clear throughout the whole palace guard and to everyone else that I am in chains for Christ."

Paul was imprisoned but used his confinement to honor and glorify God in spite of his limitations. Paul saw this as an opportunity to continue his ministry wherever he happened to be and tell others what Jesus had done for them.

I have fibromyalgia. I have limitations. While I'm no longer able to work, I am looking at my life through Jesus' eyes. I'm right where he wants me. Like Paul,

I'm encouraging others with the Lord's positive spirit. I'm living the life God has chosen for me and using it as an opportunity to minister to others. How are you responding to the pain in your life? Our actions reflect what is going on deep inside us. I have chosen faith in God for my healing. God is enough and all I need. Joy comes from God despite the pain.

Whether or not you're having a bad day or good day with fibromyalgia, look for ways to demonstrate your joy and faith to family and friends. Never allow fibromyalgia to control you. Living with daily pain and fatigue is a large part of my life now, but I will endure. I will continue going on dates with my husband. I will continue spending time with my children. I have made a commitment to attend church each Sunday, which is a day I look forward to. I will not let my symptoms limit my activities. Family and church are more important to me than my pain. Saying no is not an option. God will give me the strength to say yes to what is important to him.

The two most important choices you'll ever make are to either live for the Lord or live for the world. If your life on earth is all you have, then money, promotions and possessions will be the values you strive for. Or you can choose to be in a committed relationship with God. With him you have eternal life. In spite of fibromyalgia there is joy, peace and contentment in your walk with Jesus Christ our Lord and Savior

Fibromyalgia

Fibromyalgia is chronic widespread muscle and joint pain found throughout the body. Fibromyalgia decreases physical activity and in extreme cases may be debilitating. Fibromyalgia is more prevalent in females but found in males also. There are no two individuals that experience fibromyalgia in the same way. A treatment that works for a friend may not work for you; this also includes diet and type of exercise. It's a guessing game to find out what may help lessen fibromyalgia symptoms. You may wake up feeling well but by 11:00 AM you will feel the need to go back to bed. It's a constant fluctuation throughout the day. What was an eight or a ten on the pain scale one day will lessen to a three or four tomorrow.

Fibromyalgia is known as the invisible illness. As friends and family discover you have fibromyalgia they may say, "You look good." Be patient, the other person doesn't understand what you go through and how you feel on a daily basis. There was also a time you didn't understand fibromyalgia so take the comment as a compliment and encouragement. There are many times we can't see the pain in others as they may suffer with headaches, back pain or arthritis. So we need to also be patient as others go through their own invisible illnesses.

> Symptoms: restless legs; chronic fatigue; sleep disturbances; headache-migraine and/or tension; depression/anxiety; fibro fog-inability to think quickly, multi task, or concentrate; eighteen specific tender points where muscles are tender to the touch found at the neck, shoulders, chest, hips, knees, elbows, wrists and low back; jaw pain (TMJ); irritable bowel syndrome; sensitivity to foods, bright lights, loud noises, odors, some medications; dizziness; chronic ache and stiffness throughout the body; muscle knots

that spasm and seize up; nerves feel raw causing anxiety, irritation and frustration; premenstrual syndrome; vision problems; dry eyes and mouth; impaired coordination; weather sensitivity. If you experience any of these symptoms that may be out of the ordinary to you please contact your physician.

Cause: The cause is not completely understood and remains a mystery but there are two possible origins of fibromyalgia: One being physical trauma such as major surgery, acute illness, car accident and injury; and emotional trauma- divorce for example. Another possible cause may be genetics.

Now that you've been diagnosed you need to decide how to treat fibromyalgia. There are a few prescription drugs, check the side effects carefully and thoroughly and always find an MD, pain specialist or rheumatologist who is knowledgeable in fibromyalgia that you can sit down with and discuss your options. Supplements found at health food stores are another option as well as chiropractic or acupuncture if you choose the natural way. More treatment ideas: gentle exercise to keep muscles flexible; healthy diet; eight hours of sleep; deep breathing; lessen stress; massage; warm water therapy; pace yourself; retain a positive attitude and prayer will help decrease flare-ups. Make good use of your time when you feel good but don't overdo it. Discover the new you and accept your limitations.

Fibromyalgia affects everyone around you so sit down with your family and friends and educate them on fibromyalgia. Knowing that your loved ones understand what you are going through will help a great deal. Communicate with them what you are dealing with and that there may be life style changes. There is one last thing to comment on and that is the helpfulness of others. Once they find out that you have fibromyalgia they may have a list of ways to make you better. Thank them but also explain that you are under a doctor's care and together you are trying to figure out how to handle your symptoms.

Chapter 1

Healing

Matthew 9:1–8 Mark 2:1–12 Luke 5:17–26

Jesus was born in Bethlehem, Matthew 2:1 (NIV). Mary and Joseph's hometown was Nazareth, so naturally Jesus grew up in Nazareth. Matthew 9:1 (NIV) tells us that Jesus stepped into a boat, crossed over and came to his own town or his hometown, Capernaum. (Matthew 4:13–16 states that this move fulfilled prophecy according to Isaiah 9:1–2.)

Jesus has a reason for everything he does.

The most important reason for Jesus' move to Capernaum was to get away from the opposition he found in Nazareth. Sadly, Jesus found rejection everywhere he went. The passages of John 6:42 (NIV), Matthew 13:55–58 (NIV) and Luke 4:22 (NIV) speak of the Nazarene's rejection of Jesus. They knew who his parents were and they watched him grow up, so how can he say that he came down from heaven?

The next rejection is even more personal as it comes from Jesus' brothers, found in John 7:3–5 (NIV). This does have a happy ending because his brothers do become believers, Acts 1:14 (NIV). The resurrection probably had a lot to do with their change of heart. The Old Testament is full of rejection by the Israelites. Jesus faced a most painful rejection alone at the cross. He is rejected today in every way through schools, government, churches and hearts turning away from him.

God gave us free will to accept Jesus as our Lord and Savior or to reject him. Along the way, he knew who would become part of his family of believers. Those of us who believe were actually chosen. We were predestined before the world was created, revealed in Ephesians 1:4–5 and 11 (NIV). His plan of salvation was also foreordained. "He was chosen before the creation of the world." 1 Peter 1:20 (NIV)

It's so easy to feel down or negative because fibromyalgia seldom gives us a day off. Every hour of every day I'm dealing with a symptom of fibromyalgia. I can't remember a day since 2004 that I felt like my old self. But, if we choose to good can come from fibromyalgia. That goodness begins with knowing God chose us to be his very own. We never know where God will lead us if we would only be open to his will. Commit the matter of fibromyalgia into the Lord's loving hands and leave it with him. Don't look back. Concentrate on your future with Jesus. "I made you and I will care for you. I will carry you along and be your Savior." Isaiah 46:4 (TLB)

I want you the reader to look at fibromyalgia in as much of a positive light as possible. It has taken me years to get to this point. It didn't happen over night. It's been a journey and this fibromyalgia road has not been an easy one. God didn't promise me it would be. He did promise to walk with me and never leave me. That's all I need to know.

In the last couple years my life with God and fibromyalgia has been coming together. I am now more compassionate towards others who are in pain either physically, emotionally, or spiritually. I never would have had a reason to start a support group if it wasn't for fibromyalgia. Because of the support group I have four new friends in my life. I would not have been open to being God's willing servant in writing this book to honor and glorify him if it weren't for fibromyalgia.

Romans 8:28 (NIV) informs that all that happens to us is for our own good if we love the Lord. Ephesians 1:11 (NIV) sends us more encouragement: all things work together for the purpose of God's will. God doesn't make mistakes. He does all things well. Jeremiah 29:11 (NIV) explains that the Lord knows the plans that he has for us. They are plans to bless us with a future and a hope Psalm 139:13–19, concentrating on verse 16 (NIV). Jesus has all my days scheduled before any of them came to be.

By now people were familiar with Jesus. Mark 2:1 (NIV) states that he had come home. Word had gotten out that Jesus was back in Capernaum. Word spread, people heard, people came. Why? They had heard of his healing, driving out demons and Jesus' healing touch on the lepers. (If you're not quite sure about leprosy, it was a severe skin disease that was highly contagious.) I'm sure the disciples told the story to everyone they met how Jesus calmed the storm when they were all in a boat together on the Sea of Galilee. The disciples were amazed that even the winds and the waves obeyed him Matthew 8:23–27 (NIV). Many had heard of his teaching the good news and the coming Kingdom.

So many came from different directions to hear him preach that there was no room left in the house, not even outside the door Mark 2:1–5 (NIV). The Pharisees also followed Jesus to the house. They came from three different villages, Galilee, Judea and Jerusalem. Luke 5:17 (NIV)

The Pharisees were haughty teachers of the law. They tried to appear good, but their hearts were far from God. They had their own version of their made-up laws that they expected everyone to follow, including Jesus. They were so wrapped up in these laws that they ignored the scriptures. They rejected Jesus' claim to be the Messiah. They didn't understand that the Messiah was standing right there with them. Jesus had a few choice descriptions of the Pharisees, found in Matthew 23 (NIV). He calls them hypocrites, blind guides, blind fools, snakes, sons of vipers. A hypocrite is a pretender. There is no bigger hypocrite than the person who pretends he doesn't need Jesus. The Pharisees rejections of Jesus ultimately lead to them plotting Jesus' death on the cross. Mark 3:6 (NIV)

How awesome to have such caring friends, men who had faith in Jesus! The Bible doesn't tell us specifically that the paralytic had faith, nor does it mention that the paralytic asked or begged his friends to take him to Jesus, or that he went willingly. These men obviously knew the paralytic well and wanted him healed. The men thought a lot of him to take such gentle care and determination in lowering him down to Jesus.

In Bible times, houses were built of stone with flat roofs made from a mixture of mud and straw. Each house had outside stairways that led to the roof. The passage in Mark tells us that there were four who took it upon themselves to carry the paralytic (vs.3). Because it was so crowded in the house, they went up the side steps to the roof and dug their way through the ceiling to lower their friend right in front of Jesus (vs.4).

Jesus sees faith in the men carrying the paralytic in Matthew 9:2 (NIV), Mark 2:5 (NIV), and Luke 5:20 (NIV). When Jesus saw their bold belief or the faith of the four men he said to the paralytic, "your sins are forgiven."

Reread Jesus' words to the paralytic. It is the same personal message for you.

Is there someone you need to bring to Jesus just as the four men did? Is there a name or two that instantly comes to mind, someone who doesn't know the name of Jesus personally? Please be in prayer for God's direction and wisdom in reaching that person. Also pray that their heart be opened to Jesus and that they will not reject him.

Jesus chose to heal the paralytic's spiritual wounds before addressing his physical needs. Spiritual healing is more important to God than physical. Not until we're in heaven will we be completely healed. What Jesus wants for us now is to know him personally as the Risen Savior. Jesus sees our need more for spiritual good health than physical. This healing comes only from Jesus. If Jesus has healed you in the past, spiritually or physically, give him praise and glory now.

Mark 2:5 (NIV) Jesus saw their faith. It's assumed that Jesus saw the four men's faith. This would leave the paralytic spiritually crippled as well as physically crippled. If the paralytic didn't have faith before he was healed he certainly had it after his healing.

The Pharisees accused Jesus of blasphemy in Matthew 9:3 (NIV), Mark 2:7 (NIV), and Luke 5:21 (NIV). They thought to themselves, who does he think he is? Who but God can forgive sins? We read those specific words in Luke 5:21 (NIV) and Mark 2:7 (NIV)—who can forgive sins but God alone? The answer is in Isaiah 43:25 (NIV). Only Jesus blots out our sins and never thinks of them again. Jesus forgave our sins on the cross. That would be enough for us, but not for Jesus. He also removes our sins as far as the east is from the west. Jesus forgives, Jesus forgets. He doesn't remind us later of our sin. This is a good personal reminder to us not to bring up past hurts to others once forgiven. Isaiah convinces us that only God forgives sin, but it doesn't convince the Pharisees.

The Pharisees were dishonoring God and speaking falsely of him also known as blasphemy. They thought that Jesus was claiming to be God and that he was performing miracles that only God can do, according to Leviticus 24:15–16 (NIV), this was punishable by death. But Jesus is God and he proved it through his healing touch physically, but first and more important through his forgiveness of sin.

The Pharisees' accusations were not said aloud. Jesus knew their thoughts. Don't you think the Pharisees were taken aback when their thoughts were answered audibly by Jesus? Jesus knew their minds, asking, "Why are you thinking such evil thoughts? Why does this bother you? I'm the Messiah, I have authority to forgive sins, but anyone can say that so I'll have to prove it by healing this man." Jesus turns his attention once again to the paralytic. In all three Gospel accounts Jesus says to the paralytic, "Get up, take your mat and go home."

Throughout the Bible I have never seen Jesus as passive. I see him commanding, not demanding. I see him in charge of every situation. When he called his twelve disciples and said, "Follow me," they dropped everything, left their livelihoods behind them and followed Jesus. Jesus' ministry of healing physically and spiritually continued through these twelve men when he sent them out to preach the kingdom of

God and to heal the sick found in Luke 9:1–6 (NIV). When the paralytic heard the voice of Jesus, "get up, take your mat and go home," the man did just that. Notice there was no doubt in the paralytic. He heard the voice of Jesus and obeyed. Mark tells us he walked in full view of them all (vs.12). Luke 5:25 (NIV) adds that he went home praising God. For the rest of the day and the rest of his life this man had a bright life, full of hope and endless possibilities, a life full of gratitude and praise for Jesus. I like to think he continued to praise God and tell everyone he met about the wonders of Jesus. The paralytic didn't just walk home. For the first time in his life he was able to run, skip and jump with his four friends by his side. When he got home, I bet the first thing he did was take the stairway on the side of his house two steps at a time.

Everyone in the crowd was amazed. They were filled with awe and they praised God. Jesus has the power to do what we deem the impossible. Only Jesus died on the cross to save us from our sins. He thought of you and the future of mankind on the cross. I received my spiritual healing. Have you?

There is nothing and no one more important in your life than Jesus.

We can't end this chapter without learning an important lesson from the four men who cared so deeply for their friend. They showed him support, encouragement and friendship. They didn't abandon their friend.

Support groups work the same way. If there is one in your area, join. If not, start one and open your home to a few friends who have fibromyalgia or someone who lives in pain. Your group's aim is to give each other encouragement, friendship and support, share knowledge and personal experiences at each month's meeting.

We were chosen by God; we've been spiritually healed; we've been forgiven; God is in control. We have fibromyalgia. It's not our fault. We didn't purposely bring it upon ourselves. I don't know about you, but if I had a choice I wouldn't want fibromyalgia. I wish I could bring it back to the store for a refund like the pair of socks I got for my birthday. Fibromyalgia doesn't work that simply. I don't remember wishing for or asking God to fill my life with pain and fatigue. The fact is I have it. I've been diagnosed. Upon examination it's been determined. God has examined my heart. He has determined that I am his.

God works all things for our good Romans 8:28 (NIV). He works all things together for the purpose of his will Ephesians 1:11 (NIV). Only God can take fibromyalgia and turn it into an opportunity to share the gospel with others Philippians 1:12 (NIV). Ask God how you can turn fibromyalgia into a message of faith and hope for someone who spiritually and physically needs it.

Only Christ has the ability to make the paralytic and you and I into new creations. 2 Corinthians 5:17 (TLB) says, "When someone becomes a Christian he becomes a brand new person inside. He is not the same anymore. A new life has begun."

God has been very real in my trial with fibromyalgia. I have drawn closer to him and have learned to trust and depend on him more. In fact, it wasn't until I grew closer to God that I accepted my illness. I am learning to focus on God not my pain. Throughout my constant physical limitations including fatigue, traveling joint pain, back and neck muscle pain, chronic headache, depression, dizziness, jaw pain and fibro fog God was there. When I was diagnosed in 2005 I don't remember being angry with God or asking him, "Why me?" But I do remember confusion, isolation and a fear of the unknown. I thought my life was coming to a screeching halt. I'd been a Christian most of my life but I didn't realize God was using fibromyalgia to get my attention. God had my heart but he had other plans for me, his plans. God was patiently waiting, tenderly pointing me in his direction to begin a fibromyalgia ministry. Now I have a clear message to share: Jesus is the only One who is your hope in pain.

I didn't receive physical healing from Jesus like the paralytic did. It's certainly what I expected and I knew Jesus held the power, after all two little words from Jesus "Get up!" made the weak limbs of the paralytic strong and agile. I received the same gift as the paralytic, the greatest gift- eternal life. Now my life has purpose and meaning as I encourage others in their walk with God and fibromyalgia. Let's take the paralytic's example and see our lives bright, full of hope and endless possibilities; a life full of gratitude and praise to God. We are not the same anymore. A new life has begun. When you are going through a painful day with fibromyalgia who do you turn to? I pray it's Jesus.

Chapter 2

Weakness

2 Corinthians 12:8–10 (TLB)

The first five words of verse 8 read, "Three different times I begged." The "I" in the 2 Corinthians passage is Paul. He is the author of many books in the New Testament, 1 & 2 Corinthians, 1 & 2 Timothy, Philippians, Ephesians, Colossians, Philemon, Titus and Romans. Paul was imprisoned for preaching the Good News. Many of his works were written from jail. His early training in scripture served him well as an adult. This enabled Paul to advance the gospel for Christ because of his intense knowledge of God's Word.

Paul, a Jew, was born in Tarsus. He was thoroughly trained in the law under Gamaliel, a teacher of the law and a man honored by all people. Paul persecuted the followers of the Way or Christian believers. He went as far as obtaining letters from Damascus receiving authorization to bring these people back to Jerusalem as prisoners to be punished. Jesus wanted this treatment of his children stopped. Jesus knew how to get Paul's attention.

On a Damascus road around noon, a bright light from heaven flashed around Paul. He fell to the ground and heard a voice: "Why are you persecuting me?" It was the voice of Jesus telling Paul to go into Damascus. He had to be led because the light was so bright he was temporarily blinded. Paul met up with a man named Ananias who restored his sight and went on to explain that God had chosen Paul to know his will. Jesus wanted Paul to take his message everywhere. Paul was baptized and his sins were washed away. Paul was obedient. God transformed Paul into a preacher. Paul was passionate about sharing his testimony and being a witness for the Lord. He preached throughout the Roman Empire on three missionary journeys.

"Three times I begged." I wonder, is it okay, as Christians with a great faith, to pray over and over again for the same specific need?

The answer very clearly states in Luke 18:1 (NIV), "always pray and don't give up," and Colossians 4:2

(TLB), "Don't be weary in prayer; keep at it; watch for God's answers and remember to be thankful when they come." Galatians 4:4 (TLB) "God decided on the right time to send his son, born of a woman, born as a Jew," God decided on the right time to send Jesus. As Christians we pray for a specific need and rely on his timing. God works in his own way; in his own time. No one can rush him or run ahead of his will. The times that we find ourselves waiting impatiently rest in God, knowing he is working on fitting all the puzzle pieces of our lives together.

1 John 5:14–15 (NIV) "This is the confidence we have in approaching God that if we ask anything according to his will he hears us." As we wait for God to answer remember he sees the future. God sees the complete picture, not just our present moments. Maybe what we're praying for isn't in our best interest. He has a greater purpose in mind and he's lovingly telling us no just as he said no to Paul. God has great wisdom and knowledge. It's impossible to understand his decisions Romans 11:33 (TLB).

The scripture for this chapter is found in, 2 Corinthians 12:8–10 from the (TLB). "Three different times I begged God to make me well again. Each time God said, 'I am with you; that is all you need. My power shows up best in weak people.' Now I am glad to boast about how weak I am; I am glad to be a living demonstration of Christ's power, instead of showing off my own power and abilities. Since I know it is all for Christ's good I am quite happy about "the thorn" and about insults, hardships, persecutions and difficulties, for when I am weak then I am strong, the less I have the more I depend on him."

Verse 9 speaks to us personally. "You may say, I can't go on because of fibromyalgia," God says, "My grace is sufficient for you, for my power is made perfect in weakness."

God willingly died on the cross to save us from our sins. Without God salvation could not be found. He came to earth from heaven to rescue us and forgive us from our sin, something we could not do on our own. The same hands that were nailed to the cross are anxious to hold you close. "So overflowing is his kindness towards us that he took away all our sins through the blood of his Son, by whom we are saved; and he has showered down upon us the richness of his grace-for how well he understands us and knows what is best for us at all times." Ephesians 1:7–8 (TLB)

I find it fascinating how we've been able to wrap God's Word around fibromyalgia. Living with fibromyalgia often leaves us feeling weak. Fatigue is one of the many symptoms. We will find strength in God's Word and through Paul, who personally experienced pain and suffering, but chose to live in joy. Hopefully we'll also make the same choice.

I identify with Paul. He prayed that God would take away the "thorn." But for whatever reason God chose not to. God has chosen not to physically heal me. I'm okay with that; I have come to that spiritual growth in my life when I can say God is enough. God is all I need. We don't know exactly what Paul's thorn was. I like to pretend it was fibromyalgia. Looking into my Bible commentary I find that this thorn often kept Paul from working. It was a hindrance. It was chronic. It was debilitating. Sound familiar? The fibromyalgia that we deal with on an hour to hour, day to day basis should be a reminder to us of our constant need for God. We draw strength from

God when we are weak. If we were always strong in character, strong physically and received everything we needed on our own merit, how would God fit into our lives? Would we feel a need for God? When we admit we are weak and allow God to fill us with more and more of himself then we are stronger with him than we would be by ourselves.

To think about: Where are you in your spiritual life? Would you rather have Jesus and fibromyalgia or good health without Jesus?

Jesus is the love of my life. He's beside me during the good times; he's beside me when I'm lonely. He sees me through the tough times by supplying me with strength, wisdom and peace. That indescribable peace when Jesus speaks to my heart and says, "I have it all under control. No need to worry." God blesses me with opportunities to share his compassion and encouragement. God knows the needs of others and his timing is perfect. I just want to be obedient. He sends the Holy Spirit to nudge me when it's time to pick up the phone or write someone who's hurting. Jesus and fibromyalgia go hand in hand for me now. I have chosen to follow him and accept his will for my life. I have committed my life to him. I will not question him or doubt because he loves me and has only his best intentions for me. Without hesitation I would rather have Jesus and fibromyalgia. I trust him completely. He's kept all his promises. He has never hurt me, abandoned me or disappointed me.

Focus again on verse 9. "I am with you, that is all you need. My power shows up best in weak people." Allow God to be your focus, not fibromyalgia. Praise God and give him honor and glory for his presence in your life. He's all I need; knowing this gives me joy.

I was surprised to come across the verse in Galatians 4:15 (TLB). This verse reveals Paul's ailment or at least alludes to it. "For in those days I know you would gladly have taken out your own eyes and given them to replace mine if that would have helped me." Paul's life was forever changed by the presence of Jesus Christ on that Damascus road. Everything he penned and everywhere the Lord sent him to preach was done for the glory of God. The last thing he wanted to lose was his vision. Praise God for the gift of sight. Praise God that once you were blind spiritually you now see him clearly and what he did for you on the cross. The NIV states Paul's concern for the Galatians and asks in verse 15, "What has happened to all your joy?" (The TLB makes a clear statement that Paul had a disease of the eyes, the NIV does not. The mystery of Paul's thorn continues.)

> "It is God who arms me with strength
> And makes my way perfect
> He makes my feet like the feet of a deer
> He enables me to stand on the heights
> He trains my hands for battle;
> My arms can bend a bow of bronze."
>
> Psalm 18:32–34 (NIV)

Or to word it more personally it may read-

> God fills me with strength
> And protects me wherever I go
> God will give me surefooted
> Confidence through difficult times
> God is the Great Warrior who
> Strengthens me in times of trouble.

Are there challenges in your life? God doesn't always promise to eliminate them but he does bless us with his strength to see us through. So whatever road you're traveling on, no matter the trial or the battle you're fighting, God refuses to leave us. He walks beside us, shows us what we need to learn and gives us the strength to face our problems head on. If it weren't for fibromyalgia I wouldn't be reaching out to people in pain. God chose a different route for my life that I never would've chosen on my own. Yes, there have been trials, but I want to follow his will and he's been beside me; he's never left me.

We find in Psalm 46:1 (NIV) that nothing under his control can ever be out of control. The verse says, "God is our refuge and strength, an ever present help in trouble."

The encouragement continues in the book of Psalms, chapter 73, verses 23–26 (NIV), "Yet I am always with you, you hold me by my right hand. You guide me with your counsel and afterward you will take me to glory. Who have I in heaven but you, and earth has nothing I desire besides you. My flesh and my heart may fail but God is the strength of my heart and he is mine forever."

What a beautiful thought: Jesus holding me by my right hand. I never want to let go. Take that image with you when you are going through a difficult day with fibromyalgia. God will guide me all my life with his wisdom. Afterward he will take me to be with him in heaven. I desire no one on earth as much as God. No matter what happens, God remains. He is the strength of my heart. He is mine forever.

To fully realize the strength of God Job 38 gives us a few verses of God's unfathomable ways: "He laid the foundations of the earth. He determined its dimensions. God supports the foundations and laid its cornerstone. He decreed the boundaries of the seas as they gushed from the depths. He commands the morning to appear and causes the dawn to rise in the east and robes it in red. God holds back the stars. He ensures the proper sequence of the seasons. He shouts to the clouds and makes it rain. He imprints knowledge on the heart. He is wise enough to number all the clouds" 38:4–8, 12, 14, 31–32, 34, 36–37 (TLB). God's strength never grows weary. He's always in full supply. He's never too busy to listen to your prayers and bless you with what you need to get through another day.

If God has blessed you with strength in the past, give him glory and thank him. He'd love to hear from you.

Isaiah 40:29–31 (TLB) "He gives power to the tired and worn out, and strength to the weak. Even the youths shall be exhausted, and the young men will all give up. But they that wait upon the Lord shall renew their strength. They shall mount up with wings like eagles, they shall run and not be weary; they shall walk and not faint."

Philippians 4:13 (TLB) "for I can do everything God asks me to with the help of Christ who gives me the strength and power." We are never given more than we can handle.

"Jesus is the Father of our Lord Jesus Christ, the source of every mercy and the one who so wonderfully comforts and strengthens us in our hardships and trials" are just a few of Jesus' wonderful attributes in 2 Corinthians 1:3–5 (TLB) and (NIV). Why does He comfort and strengthen us in our hardship and trials?

"So that when others are troubled, needing our sympathy and encouragement, we can pass on to them this same help and comfort God has given us. You can be sure that the more we undergo sufferings for Christ, the more he will shower us with his comfort and encouragement." God gave each of us a message: our testimony, to share. Don't keep it to yourself.

Psalm 138:1–3 (TLB) "Lord, with all my heart I thank you. I will sing your praises before the armies of angels in heaven. I face your Temple as I worship, giving thanks to you for all your loving kindness and your faithfulness for your promises are backed by all the honor of your name. When I pray you answer me and encourage me by giving me the strength I need."

Paul was happy about his thorn because it forced him to depend on God in his weakness. Paul begged God three different times to make him well again and remove his thorn. God said no. Paul accepted his thorn and realized it was for Christ's good.

Mark 15:15–20 (TLB) reveals to us that Jesus was flogged with a leaded whip. The Roman soldiers took him and dressed him in a purple robe, made a crown of sharp thorns and put it on his head and mocked him yelling, "Hail, Hail, King of the Jews." He was then struck on the head with a staff and spat upon. This Man, innocent of any crime, was then led away to be crucified. Jesus endured unspeakable torture and literal thorns shoved down on his head by angry soldiers. Why? Read the following verse:

"Jesus never sinned, never told a lie, never answered back when insulted; when he suffered he did not threaten to get even; he left his case in the hands of God who always judges fairly. He personally carried the load of our sins in his own body when he died on the cross, so that we can be finished with sin and live a good life from now on, for his wounds have healed ours!" 1 Peter 2:22–24 (TLB)

Thank God now for what he has blessed you with. Has he answered your prayers, protected you, given you strength, comforted you, blessed you with patience? Never take God's gifts or blessings lightly. Be grateful in praise and worship. Has he saved you from your sin? Allow God's blessings to draw you closer to Him.

Chapter 3

Nourishment

Matthew 4:1–4 (TLB)

"Then Jesus was led into the desert by the Holy Spirit to be tempted there by Satan." Jesus was not alone in the wilderness. This was no coincidental meeting. This did not occur without the Father's knowledge and understanding. We learn about Jesus' strength and character in how he resisted the devil.

During the time Jesus spent on earth, he was completely human. So after 40 days of fasting he naturally became hungry. Satan took this opportunity to tempt Jesus, thinking that Jesus was weak and would give into his request. He told Jesus to turn stones into loaves of bread. Satan said, "It will prove you are the Son of God." But Jesus told him no in verse 4, the scriptures (Deuteronomy 8:3) tell us that bread won't feed men's souls; obedience to every Word of God is what we need. By overcoming the devil Jesus proved he indeed is the Son of God. Jesus not only wrote the Bible through many authors, he also obeyed the Word and used it to oppose Satan.

"Be careful-watch out for attacks from Satan, your great enemy. He prowls around like a hungry, roaring lion, looking for some victim to tear apart. Stand firm when he attacks. Trust the Lord; and remember that other Christians all around the world are going through these sufferings too" 1 Peter 5:8 (TLB). Satan is also described as crafty and disguised as a serpent in Genesis 3:1. The serpent tempts Adam and Eve and wins this battle of wits by twisting God's word into lies. Our best defense is found in Ephesians 6:10–11 (TLB), "I want to remind you that your strength must come from the Lord's mighty power within you. Put on all of God's armor so that you will be able to stand safe against all strategies and tricks of Satan."

Moses, writer of the book of Deuteronomy, found in the Old Testament speaks to the Israelites, telling them if they obey all the commandments they will live and multiply and will go in and take over the land promised to their fathers by the Lord. Moses explains how the Lord humbled them by leading them through the desert for 40 years, testing them to see how they would respond and whether or not they would really obey God. God let them go hungry and then fed the Israelites with manna. He did it to help them realize that food isn't everything and that real life comes by obeying every command of God. God wanted the Israelites to entrust their lives to him. That's what God wants from each of us as well. Like any relationship it takes work and a daily commitment.

Never allow temptation to control you. When tempted, use God's Word as Jesus did and the Holy Spirit will direct you to verses that can speak to you and help you if you are open to his leading. Submit to God and Satan will flee.

God's Word is nourishment for our souls. Deuteronomy 8:3b (TLB) says, "Food isn't everything and real life comes by obeying every command of God." Matthew 4:4 echoes the Old Testament-"Man does not live on bread alone, but on every word that comes from the mouth of God."

Our world is full of financial distress, job layoffs, rumors of war, nuclear missiles and health care changes. The list of governmental worries is endless. Yet there are two unwavering constants. Both go hand in hand. It is God and his Word. Both are dependable, never changing. No matter what happens next, God knows our future. God and his Word are eternal. Lean on God, read his Word and find comfort and peace.

Mark 13:31 (NIV) "Heaven and earth will pass away but my words will never pass away."

God's Word doesn't exist as a history lesson or general information. God wants us to be transformed. When you read God's Word you find out about his character, how he wants you to live a life that mirrors his. Praying and reading the Bible draw us to a close and intimate relationship with our Lord and Savior. God's Word changes our attitudes, direction and behavior. It shows us right from wrong. We find a new purpose in our life. His Word shows us how to live for him and serve him. His Word shows us what we're not and where we need to be more Christ-like. We turn from living selfish lives to lives that honor God. You never know what time in the

Word will bring. It's too great a risk to miss even for one day.

"For the word of God is living and active. Sharper than any double-edged sword, it penetrates even to dividing soul and spirit, joints and marrow; it judges the thoughts and attitudes of the heart." Hebrews 4:12 (NIV)

"For no prophecy recorded in Scripture was ever thought up by the prophet himself. It was the Holy Spirit within these godly men who gave them true messages from God." 2 Peter 1:20–21 (TLB)

"All scripture is God-breathed and is useful for teaching, rebuking, correcting and training in righteousness, so that the man of God may be thoroughly equipped for every good work." 2 Timothy 3:16–17 (NIV)

The authors of the 66 books of the Bible, written over 1500 years by more than 40 authors, wrote what God wanted them to write. Just as we put our trust in God we can also trust scripture because it came from God. God was in control of putting the Bible together.

In Genesis we learn of God's majestic power to

create the beauty of the world around us. But by chapter 3 sin has already entered this paradise and by chapter 6 the Lord sees how corrupt his world has become and he does away with all humanity except Noah and his family who were the only ones left still worshiping God.

Moses appears on the scene in Exodus and is chosen by God to lead his people the Israelites out of slavery. They miraculously cross a divided Red Sea and are saved. Yet this nation, chosen to bring salvation to the world, does nothing but complain. The Israelites dealt with God's punishment by wandering for 40 years in the desert. Also in Exodus we receive God's wise guidance in the Ten Commandments.

The Israelites' story continues through the book of Joshua when they finally arrive in the Promised Land. Joshua and Caleb are the only two out of more than a million people to actually enter the Promised Land. A beautiful verse 24:15 (NIV) towards the end of the book reads, "As for me and my household, we will serve the Lord." The Living Bible words this verse as a decision that needs to be made, "If you are unwilling to obey the Lord, then decide today whom you will obey."

2 Samuel records the history of David's reign over Judah and Israel. Because of his sin with Bathsheba we learn there are consequences. But God is always ready to forgive.

Esther became queen, risked her own life to save her people, the Jews, from death. She believed that she had "come into this royal position for such a time as this."

In Job we read Job is tested. Everything is destroyed yet Job does not give up on God.

The Book of Psalms blesses us with comfort and praise to God through our trials.

Proverbs teaches us wisdom.

Isaiah Chapter 7 tells us to stand firm in our faith or we will not stand at all. Chapter 12 states that God is our salvation.

In Jonah we learn that it is better to obey God than to run from him.

Matthew, Mark, Luke and John each tell the story their way about Jesus' birth and ministry. Jesus is the Messiah, the Savior of the world.

Acts fascinates us with the beginnings and growth of the church.

Philippians is filled with joy in knowing the Lord.

Revelations, the last book of the Bible, reveals to us the future and hope we have as believers that one day soon we will be with Jesus in heaven and what happens to those left behind.

Romans 10:8–10 (NIV) "The Word is near you, it is in your mouth and in your heart, that is, the Word of faith we are proclaiming: that if you confess with your mouth, Jesus is Lord, believe in your heart that God raised him from the dead, you will be saved."

Have you received God's gift of salvation?

If you said yes, your future is secure in the arms of the Savior. He is in your life, your sins are forgiven, and you are his child. You will spend eternity in heaven with God. Each day is an adventure when spent with him.

If you answered no, remember sin separates us from God and because of that separation we can't experience God's love, forgiveness and abundant and eternal life. The most important decision of your life is to be ready for the next one. "If you confess with your mouth, 'Jesus is Lord' and believe in your heart that God raised him from the dead, you will be saved," Romans 10:9 (NIV) it's that simple, come just as you are. "For the scriptures tell us that no one who believes in Christ will ever be disappointed!" Romans 10:11 (TLB)

Growing up in a Christian home is where my testimony begins. It was my parents who made sure we were a family attending church each Sunday. My parents' salvation was important to them because it was important to their parents and their parents before them. I am the result of that generational faith. I followed my parent's example and made sure that my children also received Jesus as their Savior. Jesus has always been a part of my life even before I asked him into my heart at the age of 12 away from my parents for the first time and homesick. Jesus filled that void in my life and assured me that I would never be homesick again.

Jesus didn't give into Satan's temptation. What a prime example he is in our own lives. Be on guard and watchful of Satan's attacks. Rely on Jesus' strength and read his Word.

Is Satan trying to tempt you in any way? Be in prayer immediately and ask God to take away this temptation and to give you strength to say no. Jesus had the power to stand up to the devil. He resisted his every temptation. He will certainly help you. Hebrews 4:15 (TLB) tells us that Jesus understands our weakness. He had the same temptations we did but he never gave into them and sinned.

Jesus wants us living for him not the world. He doesn't want us to be misled by the worlds way, so don't be deceived that your job, a new car, a large bank account will complete your existence on earth. Jesus wants us to be good stewards of what he blesses us with. A relationship with Jesus gives us true and lasting happiness. Jesus wants us to show the people that we work with or anyone we encounter that we belong to Jesus. "Don't copy the behavior and customs of this world, but be a new and different person with a fresh newness in all you do and think. Then you will learn from your own experience how his ways will really satisfy you," Romans 12:2 (TLB). I have learned that I need the spiritual stability of the Lord not the false securities the world offers.

Isaiah 55:2 (TLB), "Why spend your money on foodstuffs that don't give you strength? Why pay for groceries that don't do you any good? Listen and I'll tell you where to get good food that fattens up the soul."

Isaiah 55:3 (TLB), the first 3 words of verse 3 tell us where we find the food that fattens our souls, "Come to me." We find in this lesson just like the first, God is more interested in our spiritual well-being than physical, or in this case, physical satisfaction through food. God offers us nourishment that feeds our souls, his free gift of salvation.

I wonder what Jesus ate? What food did his mother Mary prepare for him while he was growing up? What foods did the disciples and Jesus consume during their earthly ministry? Jesus says in John 4:34 (NIV), "My food is to do the will of him who sent me and to finish his work." John 6:35 (NIV), "I am the Bread of Life. He who comes to me will never go hungry and he who believes in me will never be thirsty." Jesus promises to satisfy our spiritual hunger as well as our thirst found in John 4:14 (MSG), "Anyone who drinks the water I give will never thirst-not ever. The water I give will be an artesian spring within, gushing fountains of endless life." After reading these verses it isn't important what Jesus actually ate. Jesus had a healthy diet but food wasn't his priority. Our decisions need to follow his example and that begins at the grocery store. Before you put that bag of chips in your cart, stop and pray, "Jesus will you be happy I'm eating this?" Don't bring anything home from the grocery store that will have any control over you. The less sugar and snacks you feed your body the less you will crave it. "I can do anything I want to if Christ has not said no, but some of these things aren't good for me. Even if I am allowed to do them, I'll refuse to if I think they might get such a grip on me that I can't easily stop when I want to. For instance, take the matter of eating. God has given us an appetite for food and stomachs to digest it. But that doesn't mean we should eat more than we need. Don't think of eating as important, because some day God will do away with both stomachs, and food." 1 Corinthians 6:12–13 (TLB)

I have personally found sugar, aspartame, food colorings, and caffeine to cause a flare up. But I've never had a flare up when my diet was consistent in fresh fruits, vegetables, plenty of water, whole grains, protein, cheese and yogurt. Since fibromyalgia is so individualized your body will tell you what to stay away from. Always consult your doctor if you have any question on diet and nutrition.

1 Corinthians 6:19 (TLB) "Haven't you yet learned that your body is the home of the Holy Spirit God gave you and that he lives within you? Your own body does not belong to you. For God has bought you with a great price. So use every part of your body to give glory back to God because he owns it." Be careful how you feed, use, and maintain your body. May your exercise program and diet plan be done for God's glory.

Romans 14:17–18 (TLB) "For after all, the important thing for us as Christians is not what we eat or drink but stirring up goodness and peace and joy from the Holy Spirit. If you let Christ be Lord in these affairs God will be glad and so will others."

Chapter 4

Joy

Matthew 1–2; Luke 2

Jesus loves you so much that from the beginning of time his birth and sacrifice on the cross were planned to the last detail. There were no mistakes, no surprises. "His unchanging plan has always been to adopt us into his own family by sending Jesus Christ to die for us. And he did this because he wanted to." Ephesians 1:5 (TLB)

God sent out Jesus' birth announcements out early. According to Old Testament prophecy- history written in advance, "Bethlehem, a small Judean village, will be the birthplace of my King who is alive from everlasting ages past!" Micah 5:2 (TLB)

God chose Mary, a young woman of great faith and highly favored by God. She questioned God for a brief moment then accepted the Lord's will for her life-to give birth to the Holy Son of God. Mary was engaged, not married to Joseph. Joseph, a carpenter, was a man of stern principle and upon hearing Mary's news decided to silently break the engagement. He did not want to publicly disgrace her. The same angel Gabriel, who brought the good news of Jesus' conception to Mary, persuaded Joseph in a dream.

God's plan was now in full motion. Caesar Augustus, a Roman Emperor, decreed that a census should be taken throughout the nation. Everyone was required to return to his ancestral home for registration. Joseph was a member of the royal line of King David. Mary and Joseph traveled from Nazareth to Bethlehem, the town of David.

The long awaited King was finally here after many generations long before had read and heard about. Mary and Joseph named him Jesus for he shall save his people from their sins. This will fulfill prophecy from Isaiah 7:14 (TLB) that he shall be called "Immanuel" meaning, "God is with us." "For unto us a child is born, to us a son is given, and the government will be on his shoulders and he will be called Wonderful Counselor, Mighty God, Everlasting Father and Prince of Peace." Isaiah 9:6 (TLB)

Mary tenderly wrapped Jesus in a blanket and laid him in a manger because there was no room for them at the inn. Mary's incredible love that enveloped her as she gazed upon Jesus for the first time must've been indescribable.

An angel appeared to the shepherds. They brought the most joyful news ever announced and it is for everyone: "The Savior, the Messiah, the Lord has been born tonight in Bethlehem." Suddenly the angel was joined by a host of others praising God. They sang, "Glory to God in the highest heaven and peace on earth for all those pleasing him." The shepherds could hardly contain their excitement and joy and went to see the wonderful event that had happened. They ran (wouldn't you?), to the village and found this little family of three and saw the Christ Child. The shepherds told everyone what had happened and what the angels had said praising God.

At the same time astrologers came from eastern lands. A star appeared to them standing over Bethlehem. "Their joy knew no bounds." Entering the house where the baby and Mary were they threw themselves down before Jesus worshipping. They presented their gifts, gold, frankincense and myrrh.

As required by the Law of Moses Jesus' parents took him to Jerusalem 8 days later to present him to the Lord. Simeon, a Jerusalem resident, was in the Temple. He was a good man, very devout, filled with the Holy Spirit and constantly expecting the Messiah to come soon. The Holy Spirit revealed to him that he would not die until he had seen God's anointed King. The Holy Spirit had urged him to go to the Temple that same day Mary and Joseph arrived. Simeon took the Child in his arms and praised God.

"Lord now I can die content for I have seen the Savior you have given to the world. He is the Light that will shine upon the nations and he will be the glory of your people Israel." Mary and Joseph marveled at what was being said. Simeon blessed them but then said to Mary, "A sword shall pierce your soul, for this child shall be rejected by many in Israel. But he will be the greatest joy to others." Luke 2:34 (TLB)

"He was wounded and bruised for our sins. He was chastised that we might have peace; he was lashed-and we were healed. We are the ones who strayed away like sheep! We, who left God's paths to follow our own, yet God, laid on him the guilt and sins of every one of us." Isaiah 53:5–6 (TLB)

Jesus' presence on this earth brought joy to Mary and Joseph, the shepherds, the magi, to Simeon and to us who know him as our Savior. The birth of Jesus brings Jesus to us. The cross brings us to Jesus. The Good News is that the tomb was empty. Jesus lives. We serve a Risen Savior. Jesus' resurrection proved that Jesus is greater than any obstacle. Jesus' ascension into heaven, witnessed by the disciples, gives us joy and hope that we as believers will join him there soon. "No man has ever seen, heard or even imagined what wonderful things God has ready for those who love the Lord," refers to heaven that has been created for every believer. 1 Corinthians 2:9 (TLB)

> "There is none like the God of Jerusalem,
> He descends from the heavens in
> Majestic splendor to help you.
> The eternal God is your Refuge,
> And underneath are the everlasting arms,

> He thrusts out your enemies before you.
> It is he who cries, 'Destroy them!'
> So_____ dwells safely. (Insert your name)
>
> Deuteronomy 33:26–27 (TLB)

Jesus' thirty-three years of his earthly life he always chose to live in joy. "As the Father has loved me, so have I loved you. Now remain in my love. If you obey my commands you will remain in my love, just as I have obeyed my Father's commands and remain in his love. I have told you this so that my joy may be in you and that your joy may be complete." John 15:9–11 (NIV)

The world witnesses our Christianity. Is our countenance usually sad or down? Or do the people around us see us living in joy? If we're down all the time the world will respond with "who needs it!" A joyless Christian is a contradiction in terms of what Christ can do in us. Jesus is joy. We need to live lives that declare our faith to others so the ones God brings into our lives will see our outward joy and crave what we have. "Rejoice in the Lord always, I will say it again, rejoice!" Philippians 4:4 (NIV)

We find there is much joy in knowing the love God has for us. "I pray that Christ will be more and more at home in your hearts, living within you as you trust in him. May your roots go down deep into the soil of God's marvelous love. And may you be able to feel and understand as all God's children should, how long, how wide, how deep and how high his love really is; and to experience this love for yourselves, though it is so great that you will never see the end of it or fully know or understand it." Ephesians 3: 17–19 (TLB)

Another passage on God's immeasurable love that brings us much delight is found in Romans 8:38–39 (NIV). These verses tell us that nothing separates us from his love. "For I am convinced that nothing can ever separate us from his love, death can't, and life can't. The angels won't and all the powers of hell itself cannot keep God's love away. Our fears for today, our worries about tomorrow or where we are high above the sky, or in the deepest ocean, nothing will eve be able to separate us from the love of God demonstrated by our Lord Jesus Christ when he died for us."

The Lord has examined our hearts and knows

everything about us. He knows when we sit or stand. He knows our every thought. He knows the future so he is able to chart the path ahead of us and tell us where to stop and rest. Every moment he knows where we are. He knows what we're going to say before we say it. He precedes and follows us and places his hand of blessings on our heads Psalms 139:1–5 (TLB). Jesus is aware of all we do and say because he is omniscient and omnipresent-he is all-knowing and ever present. Wherever we are we are under the watchful caring eye of our Lord.

"How precious it is, Lord to realize that you are thinking about me constantly. I can't even count how many times a day your thoughts turn towards me. And when I wake in the morning you are still thinking of me" Psalm 139:17–18 (TLB). Every day of our lives matters to God.

"Not one sparrow can fall to the ground without our Father knowing it. The very hairs of your head are all numbered. So don't worry! You are more valuable to him than many sparrows" Matthew 10:30–31 (TLB).

"You have seen me tossing and turning through the night. You have collected all my tears and preserved them in your bottle! You have recorded every one in your book" Psalm 56:8 (TLB). God knows when we cry, he sees our trials and he hurts when we hurt.

He keeps constant watch over you as you come and go, always guarding, always protecting. God cares 24/7. Psalm 121:8

We have God's assurance that he will never forget us from Isaiah 49:16 (TLB), "I have tattooed your name upon my palm." "For we are God's workmanship, (a work of art), created in Christ Jesus to do good works, which God prepared in advance for us to do." Ephesians 2:10 (NIV)

The Man who counts the stars and calls them all by name loves me and he loves you Psalm 147:4 (TLB). "Look up into the heavens! Who created all these stars? As a shepherd leads his sheep, calling each by its pet name, and counts them to see that none are lost or strayed, so God does with stars and planets!" Isaiah 40:26 (TLB)

I hope you felt what you are worth to Jesus, how valuable you are to him from the previous verses. This much love should bring great joy in your life. But there is more: You can lie down in peace and sleep. God is keeping you safe Psalm 4:8 (TLB). Stop and think about this, God is watching while you sleep. There is no need for both of you to be awake!

Many times God you have done great miracles for me. I am always in your thoughts. Who else can do such glorious things? No one can be compared to you. There isn't enough time to tell of your wonderful deeds Psalms 40:5 (TLB). Christ's death is the measure of what you're worth. "The Son of God, who loved me, gave himself for me," "I am not one of those who treats Christ's death as meaningless." Galatians 2:20–21 (TLB)

2 Corinthians 5:15 (TLB): "He died for all so that all who live-having received eternal life from him-might live no longer for themselves, to please themselves, but to spend their lives pleasing Christ who died and rose again for them." We no longer live for ourselves but live for the Lord.

Try to look at fibromyalgia through heaven's eyes. Fibromyalgia is not forever but our life with God is forever, it is eternal. God loves you, cares for you. "Please don't assume that when you get to heaven you're on the last chapter. No! Earth was only the title page and the journey God intended for us all along is the rest of the book." C.S. Lewis

Now is the time to have fibromyalgia because of it's validity as an illness in the last twenty years. We know more today about how to take care of ourselves than those who have suffered in previous decades. There is more advanced research and knowledge on this condition than ever before. Since we have a better understanding of fibromyalgia we can pass that information to our friends and family and they in turn, hopefully, will be able to better comprehend what we're going through. These facts should give us hope and joy.

The next time someone tells you, "you don't look sick," you can respond with, "You may not see my pain but I hope you see my joy each time I speak of Jesus!"

Amidst your daily routine may your attention turn to Jesus often and may you be ever thankful for what Jesus did for you at the cross and what you are worth to him. Pray that his love will fill you with joy. There will be times that you'll need to be reminded that your life isn't about fibromyalgia and what you've lost. It's about looking to a bright future and what you can gain in your walk with him. Thank him that the long awaited King is here and has taken up residence in your heart.

Chapter 5
Forgetfulness

Genesis 37 & 39 (TLB)

The life of Joseph begins in Genesis 37 at the age of seventeen. His job was to shepherd his father's sheep. Joseph had ten older but ornery half brothers that also helped tend the sheep. Joseph told his father Jacob what his sons were up to. In other words, Joseph was tattling. No one likes a tattletale. Joseph's brothers weren't any different.

Not only was Joseph an informant, he was his daddy's favorite. Why, you ask, out of eleven sons, would Joseph have been more loved than any of Jacob's other children? Verse 3 clearly answers the question. "Now as it happened, Jacob loved Joseph more than any of his other children, because Joseph was born to him in his old age."

Because Joseph was one of the youngest Jacob gave him a special gift. A coat of many colors or a brightly-colored coat as The Living Bible describes the robe.

Early in the story, Joseph already has three strikes against him. First, Joseph was the revealer of all wrong actions by his brothers. Second, his father was more partial to Joseph than the others and number three, Joseph is the only one in the family to receive a gift from his father, a richly ornamented robe.

Joseph's brothers couldn't help but notice their father's fondness for young Joseph, and hatred for Joseph grew. Verse 4 reveals, "They could not speak a kind word to him."

The drama in this story takes a nasty turn when Joseph has a dream and proudly reports it to his brothers in great detail. Joseph said, "We were binding sheaves of grain when my sheaf rose and stood upright, while your sheaves gathered around mine and bowed down to it" (verse 6). His brothers hated Joseph all the more now that they thought Joseph intended to reign over them.

The next dream didn't help matters. "This time the sun, moon and eleven stars bowed down to me," verse 9. The Living Bible words the brother's response as "fit to be tied." Joseph's dream interpretation left him with a cocky attitude, verse 8.

The brothers had gone to graze the sheep near Shechem. Jacob sent Joseph to see how they and the sheep were doing. The brothers saw Joseph approaching from a distance. After a short discussion on plotting Joseph's demise, they decided to toss him into a pit or well and tell their father that a wild animal had eaten him. But due to a guilty conscience from an older brother, Reuben they dismissed the idea of actual murder. Upon Joseph's arrival the brothers pulled off his robe of many colors, pushed him into an empty well and sat down for supper! Their hatred and jealousy led them to do away with an innocent family member, yet they could sit calmly and eat.

During the brother's meal they noticed a caravan of traders coming from Gilead, their camels loaded with spices, balm and myrrh. They were on their way to Egypt. The brothers sold Joseph for twenty shekels of silver and he went to Egypt with them.

Did the caravan of traders just "happen" to come by?

The gruesome tale continues. The brothers slaughtered a goat, dipped its blood onto the prized robe, and took their lies and deception to their father. Their father mourned the loss of his son for many weeks, believing the delusion that his son had been devoured by a wild animal.

Meanwhile, back in Egypt, the traders sold Joseph to Potiphar, an officer of the Pharaoh the king of Egypt. Potiphar was captain of the palace guard, the chief executioner.

Joseph's story picks up again in chapter 39. The Lord greatly blessed Joseph in the home of his master, Potiphar, so that everything he did succeeded. Soon Joseph was put in charge of the administration of Potiphar's household and all of his business affairs. Potiphar didn't have a worry. Oh, by the way, Joseph was a very handsome man, verse 6.

Potiphar's wife began noticing Joseph and made eyes at him, suggesting that he sleep with her. Joseph refused; after all, Potiphar trusted Joseph with everything he owned. He couldn't do such a wicked thing. It would be a great sin against God. But she kept on with her flirtation. Her advances turned into a nasty scheme. She grabbed Joseph by the sleeve and demanded "sleep with me.!" (Verse 12) Joseph tore himself away but as he did his robe slipped off and she was left holding it as he fled. She began screaming to her servants, "Look, my husband brought this Hebrew slave to insult us." She kept Joseph's robe beside her and told her husband when he came home. Potiphar burned with anger and put Joseph into prison.

If only Joseph's brothers could see him now. They would be quite happy he was in jail. Were they happy for the duration of Joseph's absence? Guilt can really wear a person down. Genesis 42:21 (TLB), "Speaking among themselves, they said, this has all happened because of what we did to Joseph long ago. We saw his terror and anguish and heard his pleadings, but we wouldn't listen." In our reading of God's Word we haven't come across a word of discouragement from Joseph. He has never once questioned God, "Why me?"

Why am I telling you this story? What could I be leading up to? The answer awaits us in the time Joseph was imprisoned. The Lord was always with Joseph. Even in prison the Lord has not left Joseph's side. The Lord granted him favor with the chief jailer. The jailer soon handed over the entire prison administration to Joseph so that all the prisoners were responsible to Joseph. The Lord was with him so everything ran smoothly. Genesis 39:21–23 (TLB)

Remember those dreams Joseph had as a teenager? Well, he's back interpreting them again but this time for a baker and wine taster for the king of Egypt. It seems the king had a temper tantrum and threw them both in prison. They each had a dream but didn't understand their meaning. But Joseph understood and explained according to Genesis 40:8 (TLB), "interpreting dreams is God's business." Notice how Joseph gives God the glory. He knew he wouldn't be where he was spiritually without God's wise counsel.

Joseph told the wine taster that the three branches in his dream meant three days. Within three days Pharaoh is going to take you out of prison and give you back your job, verse 13. "Please have some pity on me when you are back in his favor and mention me to Pharaoh and ask him to let me out of here, I am innocent and don't deserve to be here, " verses 13–14.

Pharaoh's birthday came three days later and he

sent for his wine taster who was restored to his former position. He forgot all about Joseph's plea.

Have you ever forgotten anything really important? Does it happen more and more often? Do you grow impatient with yourself? Does your family? Forgetfulness is all part of the wonderful symptom of fibromyalgia. I'm being sarcastic; it's not wonderful at all. I can be having a conversation with someone and forget the simplest words. Then I try to explain or describe the forgotten word and embarrassment often ensues. Talk about a struggle. Only another person with fibromyalgia truly understands and will help you fill in the blanks.

I connected with the wine taster. If it had been me would I have remembered to tell Pharaoh about Joseph's release from jail? If I hadn't written it down and kept it in my back pocket or in Bible times tucked it inside the belt of my tunic I would've forgotten. I feel bad for Joseph—the waiting must've been torture. Not until two years later does the wine taster remember and Joseph is released, Genesis 41:9. We can only guess how this made the wine taster feel. "Today I remember my sin," the TLB. "Today I am reminded of my shortcomings," (NIV). "I remember my faults," Nelson Study Bible. The same God who granted Joseph success in everything he touched was with Joseph in prison and in freedom. Joseph didn't doubt God. Our fibro fog will never cause us distress as devastating as forgetting a future ruler in prison. Being forgotten only happened once to Joseph. But for those of us with fibromyalgia, forgetfulness is 24/7. If you're having trouble remembering or concentrating I find keeping a to-do list and prioritizing that list really helps me stay focused on the tasks at hand, no matter how small. Don't forget to schedule time for fun or relaxation. Don't put yourself down if you don't get everything done from your list. There is always tomorrow or even next week. The need to feel productive will remain. Always remind yourself what you still can do and what you accomplish throughout the day.

Fibro fog, our forgetfulness, is not intentional. But did you know that God's forgetfulness is? When we sin, we ask for forgiveness and God forgets all about it. In Hebrews 10:17 (TLB), God promises, "I will never again remember their sins."

Our Bible story has a happy ending. Pharaoh has

a dream. Joseph, now age thirty, is brought out of the dungeon and is asked to interpret the dream. Joseph's reply found in Genesis 41:16, "I can't do it by myself but God will tell you what it means." Joseph never missed an opportunity to give God honor and glory. Joseph told Pharaoh that God is telling you through the dream that there will be 7 years of prosperity and 7 years of famine. Not only did Joseph tell Pharaoh what his dream meant, he gave him suggestions on how to handle the next 14 years so there would be enough to eat. Pharaoh appointed Joseph in charge of the entire project.

Jacob hears there is grain to purchase during the famine and sends his 10 sons to Egypt to buy grain. Remember Joseph's first 2 dreams that infuriated his brothers? Well, they came true. The 10 brothers came to Joseph not recognizing him and bowed down to him. They were given enough food to eat and we find Joseph's forgiveness towards his brothers in Genesis 50:19–21 (TLB). Joseph told them, "Don't be afraid of me. Am I God, to judge and punish you? As far as I am concerned, God turned into good what you meant for evil, for he brought me to this high position I have today so that I could save the lives of many people. No, don't be afraid. Indeed, I myself will take care of you and your families." And he spoke very kindly to them, reassuring them.

God ordained Joseph to save the lives of many from famine and reunited him with his family. Psalms 105:16–17 (TLB), God called for a famine on the land of Canaan, cutting off its food supply. Then he sent Joseph as a slave to Egypt to save his people from starvation. Only God could've turned a shepherd boy into a ruler of Egypt. "And we know that all that happens to us is working for our good if we love God and are fitting into his plans." Romans 8:28 (TLB)

Still think the caravan of traders just happened by? Jesus knows every circumstance and detail of our lives just as he knew Joseph's. Everything happens as Jesus plans it. Jesus is surprised by nothing. There is comfort in knowing we walk beside the One who is in control. The ten brothers meant to harm Joseph but Jesus used their evil and turned it into his good. Trust Jesus, he can do the same for you.

Chapter 6

Forgiveness

Ruth 1–4 (TLB)

Ruth 1:1 states, "In the days when the judges ruled" are seven words that give a background to our story. Ruth takes place in a dark time for Israel. Everyone did as they pleased. They were living selfish, sinful lives apart from God. Naomi maintained her commitment and obedience to God during this time. The judges mentioned were God's servants who brought God's teaching to a corrupt society. Judges 2:16–18 tells us that Israel was faithful to God as long as the judge lived but went back to their old sinful ways when the judge died.

Naomi, her husband Elimelech and their two sons, Mahlon and Chilion—meaning Sickly and Failing respectively—settled in the country of Moab due to a famine in the region of Bethlehem. Elimelech died, which left Naomi with her two sons. The Moabite women that Mahlon and Chilion chose as their wives were Orpah and Ruth. They stayed together as a family for ten years when, sadly, the aptly named Mahlon (Sickly) and Chilion (Failing) died. The Bible doesn't refer to a time period when Naomi would've mourned. Naomi was without any male member of her family to care for her. She knew she was destined to poverty so I doubt she wasted much time in making plans for her future.

Naomi had heard that the Lord had blessed his people by giving them crops again, so she decided to return to Israel with her two daughters-in-law.

On their journey, Naomi told Orpah and Ruth to return to their mother's house. "May the Lord reward you for your faithfulness to your husbands and me. May he bless you with another happy marriage." They all wept and said, "No, Naomi, we want to go with you to your people." Naomi replied that it was better to return to their families since she had no younger sons to be their husbands. In Bible times, God made sure widows were taken care of. If a man's brother died without a son, the widow would marry the brother. The first son she bore to him would be counted as the son of the dead brother so that his name would not be forgotten Deuteronomy 25:5–6 (TLB). This was not the case for Naomi. She not only lost a husband and two sons there is no mention of existing brothers-Naomi was on her own.

Orpah kissed her mother-in-law goodbye and returned to her childhood home. Ruth insisted on staying. "Don't make me leave you for I want to go wherever you go, live wherever you live, your people will be my people and your God shall be my God, may the Lord do terrible things to me if I allow anything but death to separate us." Ruth wasn't raised to follow God. Through her relationship with Naomi Ruth grew to love the Lord and was willing to follow the Lord's leading. Naomi must've been a faithful follower of God in the ten years she spent with her young family. Ruth saw that belief in Naomi and wanted to follow her and her God. Naomi probably kept scripture passed down from generations in her heart. "Love the Lord your God with all your heart and with all your soul and with all your strength. These commandments that I give you today are to be upon your hearts. Impress them on your children.

Talk about them when you sit at home and when you walk along the road, when you lie down and when you get up. Tie them as symbols on your hands and bind them on your forehead. Write them on the doorframes of your houses and on your gates." Deuteronomy 6:5–9 (NIV)

Naomi could not change Ruth's mind, so they continued on to Bethlehem. The city was excited at their arrival. They couldn't believe it could possibly be Naomi. She told the townspeople not to call her Naomi, but "Mara" meaning "Bitter." "I left here full with a family, a husband and two sons and the Lord has brought me back empty."

The two women arrived at the beginning of the barley harvest. Ruth asked Naomi if she could go to the field and glean the free grain left behind by the reapers. Deuteronomy again reveals to us God's love and compassion for the widows. In 24:19–22 (TLB) the gleaning law was intended to help the poor, orphans and widows. If a sheaf was forgotten, olives found on the ground or grapes under the vine the reaper was not to go back for it; the Lord your God will bless and prosper all you do. Naomi granted Ruth permission and said, "Go my daughter."

The field that Ruth found herself in belonged to Boaz. Boaz asked the foreman of the fields who the young woman was. The foreman replied that it was the girl from Moab who came back with Naomi. Boaz welcomed Ruth and encouraged her to stay in his field and no one else's. She thanked him warmly. When Ruth returned to Naomi with an overabundance of food she told of the kindness and generosity that Boaz showed her. Naomi cried excitedly, "That man is our close relative (of Elimelech); he is one of our kinsman-redeemers." Ruth 2:20 (NIV) A kinsman-redeemer or close relative was a man of wealth that could financially support another family and bear their responsibilities. God had been watching out for Naomi and Ruth. He was behind the scenes directing, caring and providing for these two women.

Naomi thought it was time for Ruth to find a husband and be happily married. Naomi may have been the first match maker in recorded history. The man she was thinking of was Boaz. Boaz was a good man. His words were sensitive to his employees and to Ruth. He was kind to Ruth in allowing her to glean his fields. Boaz protected Ruth by telling the other men to leave her alone. Following Naomi's instructions, according to 3:1–4, Ruth approached Boaz at night, lying at his feet which signified an act of yielding, submitting or surrendering to Boaz. In return Boaz would have to decide if he would marry Ruth. When Boaz awoke Ruth said, "You are my closet relative according to God's law, make me your wife." Boaz was touched by the kindness Ruth had showed Naomi. He knew she had put aside her own personal desires so that she could give Naomi an heir by marrying him.

Boaz married Ruth and she gave birth to a son. They named him Obed. He was the father of Jesse and grandfather of King David and an ancestor in the lineage of our Messiah, Jesus.

The book of Ruth is a good example of how we are to love, care and support each other as families. Jesus created us to need and want him. We can't handle life on our own. We need friends and family, we have a strong desire to connect with others. Deep inside us is a craving for Jesus and a hunger to have close relationships with friends and family. A large part of life is creating relationships. What we don't see in Ruth is that relationships can be complicated but we can't live our lives alone. Learning to get along with others is challenging. Relationships begin at work, with friends or at home with family. "Make every effort to live in peace with all men and to be holy; without holiness no one will see the Lord. See to it that no one misses the grace of God and that no bitter root grows up to cause trouble and defile many." Hebrews 12:14 (NIV) Families are a gift from God. He wants us to honor them. It's the responsibility of the family to include God in their home. This spiritual example will impact many around them.

Ruth chose to leave her own mother, father and homeland. Upon Ruth and Naomi's arrival in Bethlehem the two women didn't part ways. Ruth continued living with Naomi, caring for her. Ruth volunteered to look for food. She did all the work daily, walking the fields looking for grain throughout the harvest and never once complaining. Boaz told Ruth, "May the Lord repay you for what you have done. May you be richly rewarded by the Lord of Israel, under whose wings you have come to find refuge."

The every day work of the home-laundry, meals, cleaning, errands and bills is never ending. Does your family understand that there will be times you will not be able to help out because of your fibromyalgia? Your nearest family members see your daily struggles but those outside your family unit may see you from the outside only. Fibromyalgia is internal. We may look fine through their eyes because we are suffering from an invisible illness.

Ask parents or siblings if you have time to think about the situation they have asked of you before making a final decision because of your personal health issues. Show them support and understanding in their circumstance but then ask their understanding in your own plight. God, who lives inside your heart, will give you the strength, wisdom and the right words to say.

To communicate to your family how fibromyalgia affects you, share with them that everyone has had a bad headache. Take that headache and place it on your neck, back, hands etc. Don't place the headache throughout your body but individually to each joint. Our days begin and end with this pain so I hope this better explains why we so often can't plan too far in advance or why we can't always get everything done around the house. Looking at the family's point of view they remember how you used to feel energetic and vibrant and now you live with limitations and they're having trouble connecting the past with the present. Remember your immediate family, spouse and children have seen a change in you, they are going through this with you whether you realize it or not. It's natural to grieve for your past life as Naomi did.

Naomi felt bitter, disappointed and grieved for her past life. Her husband, two sons, home and everything familiar were gone. Naomi felt a burden for Orpah and Ruth's well being. To go through life alone would have been too much for her to handle. Naomi didn't realize that God had a plan. He was going to supply all her needs, and he started with Ruth accompanying Naomi to Bethlehem. When Naomi arrived in Bethlehem with Ruth and bitterness by her side, Naomi could've remained that way but she brought God in her heart and the bitterness didn't remain. Naomi found forgiveness in God.

With Ruth and Boaz as her family she felt their love, support and strength. May you feel that as well from your own family.

Have you ever felt that your life is too much to handle? There will be times that you will need to ask for help. Don't allow guilt to infiltrate your life because of your restrictions. Are you feeling so overwhelmed with family responsibilities or family disputes that you're starting to resent it and you need to find forgiveness?

Please fill in the blanks the name or names of those people in your life that you need to bring before the Lord in prayer:

"Now instead, you ought to forgive and comfort_____, so that _____ will not be overwhelmed by excessive sorrow, (become bitter or discouraged). I urge you to reaffirm your love for_____." Verse 11 reveals, "a further reason for forgiveness is to keep from being outsmarted by Satan; for we know what he is trying to do." Satan is trying to take advantage of us. He would love nothing more than to convince us that forgiving someone who has hurt us or wronged us is not necessary. He would rather see you live in bitterness and anger. Be aware of Satan's schemes and stay on the Christian course. 2 Corinthians 2:7–8 & 11 (NIV)

We learn so much from the Bible about God's character. He is the model for our life. Jesus on the cross is the ultimate example of forgiveness. After being severely beaten, he was led out to be executed and there they crucified him. Luke 23:34 (TLB) from the cross Jesus spoke these words, "Father, forgive them, for they do not know what they are doing."

Jesus, from the cross, also looked after his mother. "When Jesus saw his mother there, and the disciple (John) whom he loved standing nearby, he said to his mother, "Dear woman, here is your son, and to the disciple, here is your mother. From that time on this disciple took her into his home."

Because God forgave us of our sins at the cross, we are to forgive others no matter the level in which they have hurt us. This is not an option. It's a command. Matthew 6:14–15 (TLB) says, "Your heavenly Father will forgive you if you forgive those who sin against you; but if you refuse to forgive, _____ he will not forgive you."

To think about: Is it easier to go to God and confess our own sins and ask for forgiveness than it is to forgive someone else's wrong against you?

We aren't condoning the sin of the person. We hate the sin but God wants us to be examples of him so that those who have wronged us will see Christ in us and they will come to know him too.

Ephesians 4:32, (NIV), "Be kind and compassionate to one another, forgiving each other just as in Christ God forgave you."

As we grow in our Christian faith we will want to be more and more like Christ. Because we have received forgiveness we will want others to experience Christ's love and forgiveness too.

Proverbs 17:9 (TLB), "Love forgets mistakes; nagging about them parts the best of friends."

Read Romans 12:17–21 (NIV) prayerfully. God's command to us in verse 17 states,"Do not repay anyone evil for evil. Be careful to do what is right in the eyes of everybody, if it is possible, as far as it depends on you, live at peace with everyone." The first four words of verse 19: "Do not take revenge." Revenge is God's job. He will take care of those who have hurt you. It would not be wise to take matters into your own hands, trust instead in God's promises. The really hard part of forgiveness comes in verse 20,"if your enemy is hungry, feed him; if he is thirsty, give him something to drink." If you see your enemy in need for whatever reason, ask God to give you strength to meet his or her needs. Pray with them. What a powerful impact this will have on mending the relationship.

The rest of verse 20 ends with feed the enemy who is hungry and give your enemy something to drink if he is thirsty for in doing so you will be heaping coals of fire on his head. According to my Bible commentary, this phrase refers to an Egyptian tradition of carrying a pan of burning charcoal on one's head as a public act of repentance. Paul, author of Romans, was using this phrase to say that we should show our enemies kindness so they will feel ashamed and turn from their sins.

Forgiveness is not forgetting. Forgiveness doesn't mean you tolerate sin. Forgiveness does not seek revenge or demand repayment for offenses suffered. God is judge and will make everything right. Jesus died for your sins and for the sins of the person you're trying to forgive. If you are living with the consequences of someone else's sin you will find the need for daily forgiveness. Matthew 18:22 (TLB) Jesus tells us that we are to forgive 70x7. The choice you have is to live in bitterness or pour your heart out to God and find freedom in forgiveness.

It's often difficult to love your family all the time. Differences in opinion, misunderstandings, feeling taken advantage of pull us apart. When we begin to pray for family and want them to know Christ as we do God will change their attitude and he will soften their heart and ours as well.

Ruth showed tremendous respect for Naomi. She was sensitive to her needs and truly cared for her mother-in-law. Naomi's example brought Ruth to believing in God. Never give up on a family member or friend who doesn't know the Lord. Who needs spiritual healing in your family? God wants everyone to come to him and believe in him. Pray for them that they will find the lessons in this book: strength in weakness; nourishment from reading God's Word; joy in knowing Jesus as their Savior and receiving spiritual healing; forgiving a person's wrong against them and forgetting it by giving it to God and letting it go. Ruth's example is to never turn down an opportunity to do good for others and to give our best for God's glory.

One of God's greatest gifts is forgiveness of sin. Psalm 103 (TLB), lists the glorious wonders God has done for you: "He forgives sin; he heals; he ransoms me from hell; he surrounds me with loving kindness and tender mercies; he fills my life with good things; he gives justice to all who are treated unfairly; he is merciful and tender toward those who don't deserve it; he is slow to get angry and full of kindness and love; he never bears a grudge, nor remains angry forever; he has not punished us as we deserve for all our sins; he has removed our sins as far away from us as the east is from the west; he is like a father to us, tender and sympathetic to those who reverence him; the loving kindness of the Lord is from everlasting to everlasting to those who reverence him; his salvation is to children's children of those who are faithful to his covenant and remember to obey him; the Lord has made the heavens his throne, from there he rules over everything there is." "Praise him for his mighty works. Praise his unequaled greatness." Psalm 150:2 (TLB)

Is fibromyalgia keeping you up and not allowing you to sleep because of restless legs, chronic pain and headache? Is there too much on your mind that you can't shut it off, relax and sleep? The normal routine of life takes us longer to accomplish our tasks. Are there not enough hours in the day and you're concerned your tasks may not get done tomorrow either?

Revisit Psalm 103 when you're trying to fall asleep. Count your blessings, name them one by one. End your list with the greatest blessing—Jesus took our place on the cross to give us a place in heaven. "In my Father's house are many rooms; if it were not so, I would have told you. I am going there to prepare a place for you. And if I go and prepare a place for you I will come back and take you to be with me that you also may be where I am." John 14:2–3 (NIV)

Jesus teaches his disciples how to pray in Matthew 6:5–13 (TLB). "Jesus instructs them to go into their room, close the door and pray to their Father who is unseen. Then your Father who sees what is done in secret will reward you. Our Father in heaven, we honor your holy name. We ask that your kingdom will come now. May your will be done here on earth, just as it is in heaven. Give us our food again tomorrow, as usual and forgive us our sins, just as we have forgiven those who have sinned against us. Don't bring us into temptation but deliver us from the Evil One. Amen."

For those of you living daily with fibromyalgia, migraines, arthritis, back pain and even depression, I hope you have opened your Bible and found encouragement in God's Word and applied it to your own personal struggle through these past chapters. My prayer for you is that this book brought you so close to God that you accepted him as your Lord and Savior.

It is possible to find faith through fibromyalgia! I believe God will use anything or anyone to bring us closer to him. He wants us to accept his gift of salvation but the gifts we receive on our spiritual birthday don't end there. He also blesses us with faith. What is faith? 1 Peter 1:8 reads, "Though you have not seen him, you love him; and even though you do not see him now, you believe in him and are filled with an inexpressible and glorious joy." Jesus says in John 20:29b, "Blessed are those who have not seen and yet have believed." Ephesians 2:8, "For it is by grace you have been saved, through faith-and this not from yourselves, it is the gift of God." We believe in Jesus even though we can't see him now! But there will be a day that we will look upon his face when we are in heaven. What a glorious day that will be!

I would like to conclude with my favorite poem. I hope you enjoy it as much as I do each time I read it. The author is unknown and taken from the book It Won't Fly If You Don't Try by Richard Allen Farmer.

Traveling Tandem

At first I saw God as my observer, my judge
keeping track of the things I did wrong,
so as to know whether I merited
heaven or hell when I die,
He was out there sort of like a president,
I recognized his picture when I saw it,
but I didn't really know him.

But later on when I met Christ,
it seemed as though life were rather like a bike ride,

but it was a tandem bike and I noticed that Christ
was in the back helping me pedal.

I don't know just when it was
that he suggested we change places,
but life hasn't been the same since.
When I had control
I knew the way.
It was rather boring, but predictable . . .
It was the shortest distance between two points.
But when he took the lead,
He knew delightful long cuts,
up mountains and through rock places
at breakneck speeds.
It was all I could do to hang on!
Even though it looked like madness,
He said, "Pedal!"

I worried and was anxious and asked,
"Where are you taking me?"
He laughed and didn't answer,
and I started to learn to trust.
I forgot my boring life and entered into the adventure.
And when I'd say, "I'm scared,"
He'd lean back and touch my hand.

He took me to people with gifts that I needed,
gifts of healing, acceptance and joy.
They gave me gifts to take on my journey,
My Lord's and mine.

And we were off again.
He said, "Give the gifts away, they're extra baggage,
too much weight."
So I did…to the people we met.
And I found that in giving I received,
and still our burden was light.
I did not trust him at first in control of my life.
I thought he'd wreck it;
but he knows bike secrets,
knows how to make it bend to take sharp corners,
knows how to jump to clear high rocks,
knows how to fly to shorten scary passages.

And I am learning to shut up
and pedal in the strangest places.
And I'm beginning to enjoy
the view and the cool breeze on my face
with my delightful, constant companion, Jesus Christ.
And when I'm sure I just can't do any more,
He just smiles and says…"Pedal!"

Epilogue

In the year 2009 I found myself unable to work due to fibromyalgia. My health when compared with 2008 or even the year before had worsened. But somewhere between the business of my every day life, studying his word and doctors appointments my love for God grew and in the midst of my struggles he became number one in my life. I love him with all my heart, soul and mind. Matthew 22:27

In spite of my loss I feel so blessed. I believe in every word of the verse from Romans 8:28, "We know that in all things God works for the good of those who love him who have been called according to his purpose." Jeremiah 29:11, "For I know the plans I have for you," declares the Lord, "plans to prosper you and not to harm you, plans to give you hope and a future." God brought this trial of fibromyalgia into my life. He promised to walk beside me never leaving me. I had a choice to make. I could live in a never ending pity party or accept God's will for my life and turn this trial into a ministry. I chose the latter.

I am actually the happiest and most content now because I know I'm where God wants me to be and that is obeying him. My prayers have become more intimate, more honest, more trusting as I have learned to lean on him. Because of my on going trial with fibromyalgia I may not feel physically stronger but I feel spiritually stronger. I've been discarding the things in my life that I once thought were important to serve him better. I don't want to imagine life without Jesus. I rely on his promises to provide, strengthen and forgive. If I lost everything I would still have his most precious gift, his gift of salvation. What I deal with on a daily basis is nothing when compared to what our Savior endured on the cross. The year 2005 was a life changing year when I was diagnosed but when you've made a commitment to follow God every year is life changing because He's molding you into his image while you are growing spiritually.

I never thought I wouldn't be able to work. I never thought God could use me to write about my experiences. I never knew that being open to the will of God could be so exciting. I always wanted to work from home. One day while sitting at my computer I realized that God had answered that very prayer. God has predestined my days. He has blessed me with a purpose. My life has a new beginning. I am a better person coming out of this trial with fibromyalgia than when I was diagnosed. I will praise him with all my heart.

The author is unknown but I live by these words:

> Lord I am willing
> To receive what you give;
> To lack what you withhold;
> To relinquish what you take;
> To suffer what you inflict;
> To be what you require.

My life and I pray your life as well can be written in one sentence: It's all about Jesus!